Intermittent Fasting

An Exceptional Manual Featuring Authentic Anecdotes
And Highly Efficient Techniques For Attaining Optimal
Weight Loss And Adopting A Healthful Lifestyle Without
Deprivation Or Strict Dieting

Spencer Preece

TABLE OF CONTENT

The Cons Of Fasting

1) It is possible that fasting could potentially impede metabolic processes.

While it is commonly argued that fasting accelerates metabolic processes, it could be posited conversely. This phenomenon occurs because as the energy is redirected away from the digestive system, the metabolism experiences an increase in energy levels, potentially resulting in a reduction of its pace to facilitate energy preservation within the body. This can be deemed a customary response. In the event that the body abruptly ceases its regular consumption of carbohydrates, it is possible for the body to perceive a deficit in nourishment, leading to the inference that sustenance is unavailable. Due to the limited availability of resources, your body will exert increased effort in storing fat. Considering the enhanced metabolic efficiency of your body, the intake of food subsequent to the fasting period will lead to a greater accumulation of calories. Subsequently, this will negate the advantages of fasting as there is a potential for weight regain upon cessation of fasting. Hence, it is imperative to seek equilibrium.

2) You may experience feelings of lethargy and fatigue.

In the initial stages of attempting fasting prior to your body acclimating to the regimen, it is plausible that you may experience a sensation of fatigue and lack of energy. This can be attributed to the decrease in both blood sugar levels and iron concentrations in your bloodstream. This can yield the equivalent outcome of diminishing the oxygen levels in your bloodstream and consequently reducing the available energy reserves.

3) It is possible that you may experience dizziness.

The physiological impact caused by the fasting may lead to dizziness due to the reduction in blood pressure. Nevertheless, this development proves to be advantageous for individuals who suffer from hypertension. It is imperative to consult with your healthcare professional prior to embarking on a fasting regimen, as the medications you are currently prescribed may exhibit heightened effects on your bloodstream as a result.

Important Considerations to Keep in Mind

One must bear in mind that during the fast, the body enhances its energy utilization efficiency and commences seeking alternative sources of fat. This can lead to a decrease in body weight. However, this also implies that your body will experience a temporary deficiency in vital nutrients. This can cause some damage.

Moreover, there exists uncertainty regarding the impact of fasting on one's metabolism. It has the potential to yield either advantageous or detrimental outcomes on your body weight over an extended duration. It is recommended that you refrain from fasting for a duration exceeding 48 hours. Intermittent fasting does not endorse extended durations of fasting. Adhere to the recommended guidelines.

In addition, it is imperative to acknowledge that fasting is not suitable for every individual. It is advisable to seek guidance from a medical professional prior to embarking on any fasting regimen. It is not advisable for the following individuals to partake in fasting:

Expectant mothers and mothers who are currently breastfeeding.

Individuals with a prior medical record indicating a cardiac arrhythmia.

Individuals who have liver or kidney impairments.

Those with wasting diseases.

Those suffering from malnutrition.

Growing children.

Adhering To The Step-By-Step Approach Of The 16/8 Method

We have previously discussed the fundamental principles of the 16/8 method, however, it is worth revisiting for a better understanding. By adhering to the 16/8 method, one engages in a fasting period lasting 16 hours, followed by an eating period lasting a span of eight hours. During an eight-hour interval, all of your meals will be provided. In addition to these individuals, it is advisable to consume ample amounts of liquids such as water, tea, and black coffee, without indulging in any solid food or adding any sugar to your beverages. Keep in mind that the 16/8 method should not be regarded as a diet; rather, it entails adhering to a specific eating schedule.

Now that you have acquired a deeper understanding of the fast, you may be inclined to commence without delay. Although this is a viable choice, it would be prudent to familiarize yourself with additional guidelines for undertaking the fast. In the following chapter, we will comprehensively discuss a systematic approach to take. We aim to provide you with instructions on how to effectively adopt the 16/8 method. Furthermore, we will also discuss the structure of a month-long timetable as you make the transition into the rapid pace.

Initiating the Process

We have extensively discussed the advantages of the 16/8 method and its relative ease when contrasted with alternative fasting methodologies. Kindly refrain from impetuously leaping into haste. Initiating a fast without proper bodily preparation may engender notable fluctuations in hormones and mood. During the initial few weeks, one may experience a sense of discomfort prior to experiencing an improved state compared to the previous condition. Therefore, in order to alleviate this discomfort, it is crucial to establish a fasting regimen and adhere to it. A fasting regimen will encompass aspects such as your objectives, designated meal times, dietary choices, and indicators that may prompt you to pause the fasting process. Furthermore, the platform enables you to capture and record personal observations pertaining to your fasting progress, as well as identify potential areas for enhancement. A fasting regimen will also assist in reinitiating your fast should you abstain from fasting for a period of several weeks or months. The plan serves as a significant affirmation of your growth and provides guidance on measures you can undertake to foster a sense of well-being during the expedient progress. Therefore, establish a fasting regimen. Many individuals prefer to maintain this as a written journal, however, alternatively, it is feasible to record your notes in an application, a spreadsheet, or publish them on your blog. It is imperative to ensure that you possess a well-defined plan and consistently update it. Once you have prepared your notebook, the following are the prescribed steps to facilitate a seamless transition into your fast.

Establishing Your Objective

Please record your fasting objectives in your journal. What is your rationale for adopting the 16/8 intermittent fasting approach? Are your motivations for undertaking this effort primarily oriented towards improving your health, addressing medical concerns, or enhancing your overall well-being? It is imperative to possess a specific rationale behind adopting the 16/8 method. Possessing an objective can effectively sustain your motivation to persist with fasting, even during challenging circumstances.

It is imperative that your objective be formulated as a SMART goal. SMART goals are goals characterized by their specificity, measurability, attainability, relevance, and time sensitivity.

Specific. While it could be argued that your intention is to improve overall health, such an objective lacks specificity. A precisely defined objective is evident and articulates the precise area in which progress is desired. Would you be interested in improving your blood glucose levels? Are you interested in shedding body weight or reducing the size of your waistline? Would you be interested in enhancing your concentration levels throughout the day? There exists a plethora of potential specific objectives from which you may opt to commence your fast.

Measurable. Your objective, regardless of its nature, ought to be quantifiable. There ought to exist a metric that facilitates the identification of one's demonstrable progress. Quantitative metrics provide a valuable means of assessing the success of your goals, but there are other intangible aspects, such as maintaining a consistently positive disposition, that can also be indicative of achievement. As long as you diligently monitor and assess the progress of your objective, it will inherently possess measurability. If your objective is to improve blood glucose levels, it is advisable to establish a specific target value to aim for on a daily basis. This number can be obtained by consulting with your healthcare provider. If your objective centers around weight reduction or size reduction, it is advisable to establish a quantifiable figure on the weighing scale or measuring tape as your target. If you aim to enhance your concentration throughout the day, it is advisable to monitor this sensation on a daily basis. A considerable number of individuals employ mood trackers as a means to assess their daily emotions. Trackers of this nature are highly suitable for intangible objectives such as enhanced concentration, increased happiness, improved sleep patterns, and so forth. When one is able to monitor their objectives, it thereby becomes quantifiable. In the event that your objectives are not being met, you will observe such deviations in your

12

monitoring, thereby indicating the necessity for adjustments. If you are successfully attaining your objectives, you may rejoice at every significant step, acknowledging each instance of progress that brings you closer to the ultimate realization of your aspirations.

Achievable. Attainable objectives are those that you can attain. If your objective entails shedding several hundreds of pounds by means of fasting, it is impractical and unattainable. A more advisable objective would be to express a desire to shed ten pounds. This is a goal that can be realistically accomplished. After achieving this objective, you may proceed to establish a subsequent goal entailing the reduction of an additional ten pounds. Attainable objectives ought not to be those of grand proportions or ones that are excessively idealistic in nature. Choose realistic goals. We have previously discussed the ineffectiveness of setting ambitious objectives. This is because ambitious objectives often resemble distant aspirations, rather than attainable tasks of smaller scale. The presence of an ambitious objective may lead to a decline in one's motivation, resulting in the frequent failure of individuals when it comes to their New Year's resolutions. So, choose achievable goals. They do not need to be effortless; they simply need to be feasible.

Relevant. Suppose that you and your closest companion, B, make the collective decision to embark on the 16/8 method together. This is genuinely beneficial as it provides you with both a sense of responsibility and a source of encouragement. However, it is important that your objectives for the fasting period differ. Your objectives should be pertinent to your individual circumstances. Hugh Jackman adhered to the 16/8 fasting protocol in his preparation for the character of Wolverine. Is it implied, then, that you ought to pursue the identical objectives of muscle development and weight reduction as him? No, he was supported by a team of trainers, nutritionists, and coaches who assisted him in achieving those objectives. It is highly likely that you do not possess such assistance. Furthermore, are you attempting to resemble the character Wolverine? Probably not. Select objectives that have personal relevance to you. Select the dimensions that are most suitable for your needs. While Friend B may express a desire to shed 20 pounds, your focus may be on improving your sleep patterns. As long as the objective remains your own, it will retain its relevance.

Time-bound. Objectives that are bound by specific deadlines prove advantageous. This does not imply that once you have achieved your objective, you discontinue your efforts. If you so desire, you may elect to cease your current endeavor, or alternatively, you have the option to either reiterate your current objective or establish a new objective to pursue. If achieving improved blood sugar levels is your objective, at what point in time do you wish to attain this? When do you anticipate attaining your weight loss objective? When would you consider your goals to be accomplished in order to enhance your concentration in the workplace?

Ideal for: Individuals who prioritize their health and desire an additional source of nourishment

This approach entails abstaining from food for a duration of 24 hours, undertaken either once or twice weekly, with no restriction on the commencement or conclusion time. You can choose to fast from dinner to dinner, lunch to lunch, etc. Provided that you fulfill the full duration of 24 hours. The remaining non-fasting days encompass customary eating patterns, mirroring one's typical dietary habits.

It is essential to diligently maintain proper hydration throughout your fast and engage oneself intellectually as a means to prevent succumbing to temptations. Following a period of fasting, it is advisable to prepare meals in smaller quantities the next day to minimize the risk of indulging in excessive eating.

This approach yields more favorable results when supplemented with consistent exercise and a nutritious dietary regimen.

The pros

One advantage of this diet is that it is difficult to make errors in following it. The sole stipulation in place entails refraining from consuming any food for a duration of 24 hours. Consequently, should one decide to cease their intake of sustenance at a specific moment, they will patiently wait until that precise time to resume their meal consumption.

The eat-stop-eat diet does not entail any limitations on calorie intake or the exclusion of specific food groups, thereby rendering it exceptionally effortless to adhere to.

The Cons

One prominent limitation of this approach is that the majority of individuals encounter a certain level of challenge in adhering to the requirement of abstaining from food for an entire duration of 24 hours. A few prevalent grievances encompass feelings of exhaustion, irritability, and migraines - although it is expected that these symptoms will gradually abate.

Extended periods of fasting also have the potential to lead to excessive consumption once the fasting period concludes, particularly in individuals who struggle with regulating their food intake due to a lack of self-discipline, a quality that is often scarce among the general populace.

The Warrior Diet, authored by Ori Hofmekler

In accordance with its title, this approach to intermittent fasting entails adhering to a warrior-like diet consisting of uncooked vegetables and fruits during the day, followed by a substantial evening meal. Based on the dietary guidelines, you have the opportunity to indulge in an evening meal (limited to a 4-hour period) while abstaining from food during the entirety of the day (within this context, fasting involves consumption of uncooked foods).

Amongst the various intermittent fasting methods, this particular approach predominantly emphasizes the selection of specific dietary options, notably those aligned with the principles of the paleolithic diet. This implies that the sustenance ought to be in its entirety and unaltered state.

The underlying concept of the warrior diet revolves around the notion that individuals should provide their bodies with the necessary nutrients based on their inherent circadian rhythms, which dictate that humans are naturally inclined to consume food during nighttime hours.

This dietary approach primarily functions by adopting a regimen of consuming wholesome foods and minimizing caloric intake. Throughout the duration of the 20-hour fasting interval (referred to as the underconsumption phase), it is permissible to consume freshly squeezed juice, a limited quantity of vegetables, and, if preferred, a small portion of protein. As a result, this typically results in a reduced caloric intake, thus amplifying the "fight or flight" response of the Sympathetic Nervous System. Subsequently, the mechanism induces the activation of lipid metabolism and amplifies physiological vigor.

On the contrary, there exists a four-hour period for consuming meals, commonly referred to as the phase of excessive food intake, which predominantly occurs during the nocturnal hours. The objective at hand is to enhance the capacity of the

Parasympathetic nervous system to facilitate the body's recovery process by facilitating relaxation and instilling a feeling of tranquility as the body assimilates and utilizes nutrients for purposes of growth and restoration.

The pros

One noteworthy aspect of the warrior diet is the provision for indulging in modest snacks throughout the fasting phase, thereby greatly facilitating the maintenance of resilience and determination.

The method also promotes the consumption of healthy and nutritious foods, which is generally good for you.

The cons

For certain individuals, complying with the dietary recommendations and adhering to food restrictions may prove challenging over an extended period of time.

The approach may have an impact on your social interactions since, as you are aware, food serves as a significant catalyst for bringing individuals together. It is possible that you may opt to refrain from attending daytime social gatherings, particularly those organized by your family and friends, so as to avoid any appearance of impoliteness due to abstaining from food consumption.

Moreover, adhering to this approach becomes challenging if one has a preference for avoiding large meals during the evening hours.

The Physiological Advantages of Adopting an Intermittent Fasting Regimen

Observing intermittent fasting can yield numerous favorable outcomes. Let us examine a few key advantages among these.

1. Weight Loss

The detailed explanation provided in the introductory chapter will now be summarized for your convenience. When transitioning into the state of fasting, your body primarily utilizes its stored energy reserves, specifically fats, as a source of energy. As the body metabolizes these energy sources, namely fatty acids and ketones, weight is effectively and effortlessly reduced.

2. Minimizing the Probability of Developing Diabetes

There are two possible justifications for this phenomenon:

1: Achieving a state of fasting effectively leads to a significant decrease in blood glucose and insulin levels. This will ultimately lead to an enhancement in cellular insulin receptivity, consequently resulting in an improvement in the rate at which glucose is absorbed. This intervention facilitates the mitigation of insulin resistance, leading to a subsequent amelioration of diabetes.

2: Fasting stimulates the secretion of the human growth hormone, which accelerates metabolic processes and facilitates lipid oxidation within the human body. As a consequence of this occurrence, one ultimately experiences a reduction in adipose tissue. Too much weight has been known to lead to increased risk of developing diabetes. Consequently, this implies that you will mitigate your risks through the practice of fasting.

3. Assists in Cancer Therapy

Fasting facilitates the production of novel immune system cells within the body. Furthermore, it plays a vital role in diminishing the activity of PKA enzyme (protein kinase A), consequently impeding the advancement of tumor cells, cancer cells, and the aging process. When the concentration of PKA enzyme is depleted and there is an ample presence of immune system cells, it results in the deceleration of cancer cell and tumor growth. Consequently, as a patient, you can have confidence in your relative safety from cancer or the absence of expedited cancer progression.

Moreover, it is worth noting that inducing a state in which dietary glucose is absent from the bloodstream can be advantageous in combating cancer. Why is that? Indeed, cancer cells exclusively rely on glucose as their sole source for metabolic processes. Due to the absence of glucose in your bloodstream, the cancer cells are effectively deprived of nourishment. Further insights into the beneficial impact of intermittent fasting on combating cancer can be acquired by referring to the available information.

Diminished susceptibility to cardiovascular ailments

It is probable that individuals who are overweight or obese are at an elevated risk of experiencing heart-related conditions such as cardiac arrests.

Given that intermittent fasting is effective for weight loss, it consequently reduces the probability of developing cardiovascular conditions when adhered to consistently.

Enhances Brain Function

The implementation of intermittent fasting has been unveiled to facilitate optimal cognitive function by inducing the proliferation of neurons. Consequently, it can be inferred that your memory is poised to witness enhancement. Researchers have also uncovered findings that indicate enhanced proliferation of neural cells following stroke or traumatic brain injury by implementing dietary restriction. Additionally, it aids in reducing the likelihood of developing Parkinson's disease and Alzheimer's, as well. Additionally, research conducted has substantiated the findings indicating that individuals afflicted with these two neurological disorders demonstrate enhanced cognitive function and generally exhibit a high standard of living.

Skin rejuvenation

Numerous dermal issues can potentially lead to a decline in self-confidence over time. Acne illustrates this point effectively. Although numerous medications and topical treatments are promoted as the most effective solutions for acne, intermittent fasting emerges as the preeminent organic remedy for this condition. This can be attributed to the presence of excess sebum and adipose tissue beneath the skin, resulting in the development of acne and various forms of facial pimples.

In addition to alleviating the level of fat in your skin, intermittent fasting facilitates the identification of dietary triggers that contribute to skin sensitivities, thus resulting in acne and other undesirable conditions. This can be accomplished by selectively consuming specific foods while abstaining from others for a period, and subsequently reintroducing the avoided foods while monitoring the distinct responses exhibited by your skin. You will acquire knowledge regarding the appropriate food choices as well as those that should be avoided.

Tips To Get Started

It is opportune to commence implementing intermittent fasting and leverage its myriad advantages. In the following segment, we shall examine several straightforward guidelines that can be adhered to in order to initiate this dietary regimen.

Establish an objective

Prior to commencing a weight-loss regimen, it is imperative that you establish clear objectives for yourself. Establishing objectives plays a vital role in all facets of one's existence, and the pursuit of a healthy diet is no exception. In the absence of a clearly defined objective, the likelihood of abandoning the dietary regimen rises, thereby diminishing one's resolve to adhere to it. Establishing a goal provides the impetus to persevere despite encountering temptations along the path. When establishing personal objectives, it is advised to employ the acronym SMART. SMART goals are an acronym that represents objectives that are characterized by being modest in scale, quantifiable, achievable, pertinent, and bound by a specified timeframe. To provide an example, if your objective is "to reduce body weight," then it is rather imprecise. When the objective lacks clarity, the likelihood of succumbing to procrastination rises, leading to a decrease in overall motivation. An illustration of a SMART objective would be, "My aspiration is to achieve a weight loss of 20 pounds within the span of six months." This goal is notably attainable, with the inclusion of a specific time frame that serves to effectively keep one focused and dedicated to their objective. Setting imprecise or unattainable objectives inevitably leads to disillusionment. An objective such as "I aspire to shed 20 pounds within a month" is not only unattainable but also detrimental to one's well-being.

Choose an Approach

Having been informed about the various approaches to intermittent fasting, it is now necessary to make a choice. Irrespective of the approach one chooses, provided that they adhere to the prescribed dietary timetable, they can reap all the advantages that intermittent fasting provides. Please respond to the following three inquiries in order to identify the appropriate approach. If the approach you choose is not compatible with your typical way of life, the probability of deviating from the prescribed diet tends to rise.

• How do you perceive or approach fasting?

• May I inquire about your typical daily routine?

• What dietary habits do you typically follow?

By responding to these three inquiries, you are able to aptly determine the appropriate approach. For example, if the concept of daily fasting is not appealing to you, then either the 5:2 diet or intermittent fasting would be suitable alternatives. Alternatively, should you typically forego breakfast and possess an aversion to consuming late evening meals, you may choose to adopt the 16:8 intermittent fasting approach. If an individual's customary dietary intake predominantly consists of processed foods and carbohydrates, it will necessitate a considerable amount of time for the body to acclimate to any form of fasting. To initiate a systematic acclimation of your body to fasting, it is advisable to gradually diminish the consumption of unhealthy foods, restrict snacking, and extend the intervals between meals. If your regular schedule is excessively busy and barely allows time for consuming three meals, you may consider adhering to the 16:8 or the 5:2 dietary methodologies.

Select a Date

After the diet selection process has been completed, it is now appropriate to commence the chosen regimen. Implementing any form of dietary modification constitutes a significant adjustment for your physiology, necessitating a period of acclimation to the new regimen. Exercise patience and refrain from hastening, as it is not advisable to embark immediately on a fasting regimen. Conversely, select a specific date and ensure that you commence the dietary regimen from the designated date. Furthermore, it provides your physical and cognitive faculties with an opportunity to acclimate to the concept of fasting. For example, if you typically consume multiple small meals on a daily basis, initiating the 24-hour protocol may pose challenges. By allowing yourself a period of ten days to gradually condition your body for the fasting regimen, you enhance the likelihood of achieving your desired outcome. One can gradually adopt a healthier diet by incorporating nourishing and wholesome meals into one's eating routine, minimizing snacking between meals, and gradually increasing the duration between each meal. Maintaining a patient and methodical approach yields success; remember this fundamental principle as you engage in fasting. Do not hastily embark upon the practice of fasting without due consideration and caution. The most straightforward approach to mitigate the risk of prematurely discontinuing a diet is by means of adequate prior preparation.

Collect the provisions

Inexperienced individuals who embark on fasting may experience a pronounced inclination to indulge in nutritionally unfavorable food choices when they conclude their fasting period. In order to resist the allure of engaging in this behavior, it is imperative that you replenish your pantry with nutritious and nourishing ingredients. Please refer to the straightforward recipes provided in this book, as well as the accompanying list of permissible foods for consumption during fasting. It will assist you in creating a comprehensive shopping list suitable for sustenance during fasting. Ensure an ample supply of zero-calorie beverages in your possession, and you will find it more convenient to manage your periods of hunger.

Discover Your Inner Drive

Discovering your motivation is crucial in maintaining adherence to a dietary regimen. If an individual lacks a compelling rationale for adhering to a diet, it becomes implausible to sustain it over a prolonged period. It is imperative to not solely rely on your personal motivation; it is pivotal to establish a robust support structure. An established system of support provides the necessary fortitude to maintain adherence to one's dietary regimen, even during periods of despondency or reluctance. Your network of support can encompass individuals within your immediate family, close friends, colleagues, and other cherished acquaintances. They will serve as a continual reminder of your objectives and the justifications for adhering to the dietary regimen. It becomes increasingly manageable if you are able to identify a companion to embark on the diet together. Having a diet companion can effectively enhance adherence to the diet while providing companionship throughout the diet journey.

Incorporate Physical Activity
Incorporate Some Physical Exercise
Include Some Physical Activity

Incorporate a regular regimen of physical exercise into your daily schedule to expedite the process of weight reduction and enhance your overall well-being. There exists a variety of exercise options available for selection, thus obviating the need to necessarily frequent a fitness facility.

There are a variety of exercise options available, including running, jogging, walking, hiking, cycling, swimming, or engaging in a preferred sporting activity. Should you desire, you may also engage in the practice of yoga and dancing.

Prioritize refraining from engaging in high-intensity physical activities within the initial two weeks of commencing this dietary regimen. The process of acclimating to fasting typically requires a timeframe of approximately 1 to 2 weeks for the human body. Considering that your food consumption will slightly decrease, it would be prudent not to exert yourself excessively. In the early stages, you may choose to engage in gentle physical activities such as yoga and fundamental core exercises that refrain from exerting excessive strain on your cellular structure. It would solely enhance your muscular well-being. To prevent the onset of fatigue, headaches, or irritability, it is imperative to abstain from excessive exertion. Additionally, strategize your meal planning in order to facilitate regular physical activity.

Prepare Nutritious Dishes

Start cooking healthy meals and avoid eating out as much as you possibly can. It not only aids in reducing your expenses for food but also guarantees that your body receives all the necessary nutrients. There is no need to allocate any time to searching for recipes as this book provides numerous uncomplicated and nutritious recipes. Examine the recipes and formulate a personalized meal schedule for yourself. After you have devised a meal plan, allocate a specific time for the preparation of your meals. Engaging in basic meal preparation over the weekend substantially facilitates the process of preparing nutritious meals throughout the week. In the process of meal preparation, it is possible to cook a large quantity of select foods, prepare fundamental ingredients, and divide the meals into suitable portions.

Keep a diary Keep a record of daily activities Maintain a written account

Adopt the practice of keeping a dietary log as a means to enhance your awareness regarding the nutritional choices you make. Please commence the process of jotting down all the sustenance you partake in, in conjunction with your fasting regimen. There may be occasions where you experience a yearning for particular foods while observing the fasting period. These sudden and unexpected cravings may manifest abruptly and without prior indication. Thus, what courses of action are available in such situations? Retrieve your journal and commence documenting all the comestibles you desire to consume. By duly acknowledging these points, you can effectively refrain from indulging in superfluous contemplation about the various foods you desire to consume.

During this process, remind yourself that you will have the opportunity to consume it at a later time rather than immediately. By engaging in this behavior, you can avoid the sensation of depriving yourself of any nourishment and redirect your focus towards adhering to your dietary regimen anew. If one continuously ponders over their upcoming meal, it is likely that they will experience an immediate sensation of hunger.

Be Patient

Should you lack prior experience in attempting a dietary regimen, it is important to recognize that your body will require a considerable length of time to adjust to these changes. Develop the skill of exercising patience towards yourself. Should you display impatience and hastily embark upon this dietary regimen, it is plausible that you might subject your body to unwarranted strain. In our fast-paced society, we are often faced with demanding and busy schedules. Therefore, it is imperative that our dietary choices do not become an extra burden or cause of anxiety. Given the flexible nature of intermittent fasting protocols, there is no need for concern. If one consciously adheres to the fasting protocol and exercises mindfulness in their dietary choices, intermittent fasting can be deemed easily manageable. An additional prevalent error to be prevented is the act of daily weight measurement. Do not anticipate any remarkable alterations in your weight within a short span of time. Have faith in the dietary plan, adhere to it diligently, and witness a notable enhancement in your overall state of wellness.

By adhering to these straightforward guidelines, one can maximize the advantages provided by this dietary regimen.

Fat Loss Forever

This protocol might be suitable for individuals who have a fondness for exercising at the gym and indulging in an occasional indulgent meal throughout the week. The Fat Loss Forever protocol is a product of the integration of the initial three protocols that were examined, namely the LeanGains, Warrior Diet, and Eat-Stop-Eat protocols. How's that so? It amalgamates the superior attributes of said three protocols.

How to Execute the Fat Loss Forever Protocol

According to this protocol, you commence your week of fasting with a cheat day, of all things. During the span of the second and first half of the third day, which amounts to approximately 1 ½ days or 36 hours, it will be imperative for you to observe a period of fasting. During the remaining duration of 5 ½ days, you have the option to employ any of the three protocols.

Benefits of Implementing the Fat Loss Forever Protocol

One primary benefit of this protocol for the majority of individuals is the opportunity to commence their intermittent fasting (IF) week on an optimal note, specifically by incorporating a cheat day. By doing so, individuals can anticipate an enjoyable event within their IF week, fostering a sense of anticipation and enabling them to begin on a positive and elevated level.

Another benefit lies in the aspect of adaptability, particularly with regard to determining the commencement of the intermittent fasting week and selecting the appropriate protocol or protocols to be employed during the remaining four and a half days of the week. With such a malleability, there is an increased probability of adhering to the prescribed procedure for a sufficiently long duration to reap its advantages.

Drawbacks associated with the Fat Loss Forever Protocol

If mismanaged, the primary benefit it offers may also manifest as its greatest drawback. This phenomenon occurs due to the absence of self-restraint, as the designated cheat day can progressively transform into a remarkable episode of overindulgence in food, ultimately resulting in an excessively high intake of calories that potentially offset any calorie deficits that intermittent fasting aims to create. Binge eating can potentially impede fasting efforts as it is likely to generate heightened hunger pangs or an intensified desire for food during the fasting intervals. Therefore, it is imperative to exercise restraint when implementing the cheat day.

Before You Start

Prior to embarking on the implementation of any of the protocols discussed within this book, it is essential that you diligently equip yourself for this endeavor. If one desires to effectively achieve their weight loss and health objectives via intermittent fasting, it is essential to address several significant aspects.

Beliefs

Your beliefs regarding intermittent fasting will significantly influence the overall quality of your chosen protocol's efficacy. If you believe that you'll have a very miserable time while as you fast intermittently, that's how you'll feel from the get-go and it won't be long before you eventually quit. However, if your conviction regarding intermittent fasting is that it presents a commendable test that you are capable of handling adeptly and will progressively adapt to, while also acknowledging that it will effectively facilitate your desired weight reduction and promote overall well-being in due course, then your encounter will not be arduous. Additionally, the probability of maintaining your intermittent fasting endeavors for a sufficient duration to observe positive outcomes will be significantly elevated.

Patience

A considerable number of individuals have achieved significant weight loss and enhanced their overall health more expeditiously through the adoption of intermittent fasting, in contrast to other conventional and widely-adopted dietary approaches. However, it would be inappropriate to assume that your experience will necessarily align with others who have undergone a similarly swift process. Every individual possesses distinct physiological attributes and lifestyle habits that can influence the pace at which they experience weight loss and improved health through the practice of intermittent fasting. Therefore, do not become disheartened if you experience weight loss at a pace slower than your anticipated rate. The crucial aspect is your ability to consistently achieve weight reduction on a weekly basis, irrespective of the relatively minor or gradual pace at which it occurs. Ensure that you assess your weight relative to your own, refraining from making comparisons with others.

Hydration

Numerous individuals tend to overlook the significance of drinking water, yet it is a fundamental factor that can greatly aid in effectively controlling hunger sensations throughout fasting intervals and enhancing vitality levels. How?

First, let us commence our discussion on hunger pangs. Are you aware that frequently, dehydration is commonly mistaken for experiencing hunger? By ensuring adequate water intake throughout the day, you may experience a notable reduction in the occurrence of hunger sensations due to the prevention of dehydration. What will remain is a genuine sense of hunger.

Regarding the topic of genuine hunger, it is noteworthy that consuming a sufficient amount of water prior to and throughout meals can contribute to a prolonged sensation of fullness, allowing one to be satisfied with the same quantity of food, or potentially even less. This is because water serves as a stomach filler with no calories. The greater the amount of water you consume, the reduced quantity of food you will require in order to experience prolonged satiety.

Quality Sleep

This is another aspect that is frequently overlooked by individuals striving to achieve weight loss. Allow me to rephrase: If an individual consistently fails to obtain adequate sleep, it is likely that their hunger pangs will intensify and they may struggle to manage their appetite during periods of fasting. In such a scenario, all of your attempts made through IF will prove futile.

What is the mechanism by which chronic sleep deprivation influences the stimulation of appetite? Inadequate sleep instigates an upsurge in the production of ghrelin, which is the hormone responsible for stimulating appetite or hunger. Increased ghrelin production directly correlates with heightened appetite and a heightened frequency of hunger sensations.

Insufficient sleep additionally inhibits the body's capacity to generate leptin, the hormone responsible for satiety, i.e., the hormone that induces feelings of fullness. A decrease in the production of leptin by your body corresponds to a reduction in feelings of satiety. Consequently, you will necessitate consuming a larger amount of food in order to experience satisfaction or a sensation of fullness.

However, attaining a sufficient amount of adequate sleep, conversely, facilitates increased leptin production and decreased ghrelin production, leading to heightened feelings of satiety and reduced feelings of hunger. That is why it is imperative to strive for an adequate amount of restful sleep on a nightly basis.

Quality sleep is comprised of two key factors: the length of time spent asleep and the level of profundity achieved during sleep. Regarding the duration, what is the requisite number of hours of sleep you require? Although numerous experts advocate for the duration of eight hours as being optimal, it is not universally applicable. Certain individuals require a duration of merely seven hours, while others necessitate a period of nine hours. What methods do you employ to ascertain the amount of sleep you require?

Please maintain a journal for the upcoming week, specifically documenting the time of your sleep initiations and awakenings, the duration of your sleep, and your overall subjective well-being throughout each day. By examining your documented records, you can obtain valuable knowledge regarding the correlation between the amount of sleep and your overall state of alertness and vitality throughout the day.

When considering the depth of sleep, there are various measures that can be taken to enhance the probability of experiencing a profound and rejuvenating sleep on a nightly basis:

It is advised to power down all electronic devices one hour prior to bedtime in order to facilitate a seamless transition into slumber upon retiring for the night.

Abstain from consuming any caffeinated beverages after 3 pm to allow ample time for the elimination of caffeine from your bloodstream before retiring for the night.

For optimal quality of sleep, it is advisable to maintain a room temperature range of 60 to 67 degrees Fahrenheit in the presence of an air conditioner in your bedroom.

Maintain a dimly lit ambiance in your room, and if the absence of light causes discomfort while sleeping, opt for the use of an eye mask.

Engage in the act of listening to delta wave binaural beats while in a state of slumber.

Optimal Strategies for Commencing Your Fast-breaking

Fasting confers numerous health advantages, as has been previously elucidated, and similarly, breaking one's fast can yield positive outcomes if executed appropriately. Prior to elucidating the optimal methods for concluding a period of fasting, it is imperative to emphasize that one may merely proceed with their habitual dietary habits. There is no conclusive explanation as to why it is imperative to terminate your fast in a particular manner. If the inclusion of this complication impairs your capacity to observe fasting, please do not fret about it. Nevertheless, if you are able to modify your eating habits slightly for the initial meal following your period of fasting, you can enhance the outcomes.

What is the significance of consuming specific food immediately after concluding a fast? When undertaking a fast, it brings about alterations in the functioning of your gastrointestinal system. Returning to the subject matter at hand, the act of abruptly resuming regular eating patterns with a hearty meal has the potential to induce gastrointestinal distress or hinder progress towards weight loss, particularly if suboptimal food choices are made. Therefore, it is imperative to prioritize the maintenance of self-care practices during the period following the termination of fasting. There are several straightforward recommendations regarding appropriate food choices upon breaking a period of fasting.

Before solid food

Consider commencing your fast with an appropriate liquid before consuming solid sustenance to enhance the potential benefits. In the event that you commence your fast by invigorating your gastrointestinal system and preparing it for a substantial meal, you will effectively restore normal function to your intestines while preventing an abrupt surge in insulin levels that could potentially heighten your susceptibility to fat storage. The enhancement of digestive enzymes can be facilitated by employing citric acid, thus providing a beneficial boost to your digestion. Apple cider vinegar functions effectively, just as lemon-infused water does.

Bone broth is an excellent secondary option to consider, and can even be regarded as a primary choice if you choose to forego the consumption of citric acid. Bone broth aids in the restoration of gastrointestinal function and offers essential electrolytes and collagen. After completing a fasting cycle, your body will exhibit a remarkable ability to efficiently assimilate a multitude of these exceptional nutrients.

Both citric acid and bone broth have the capability to prepare your body for food consumption once more and facilitate proper digestion. Following the consumption of these beverages, it is advised to allow a period of 15-30 minutes before partaking in the consumption of solid nourishment in order to achieve optimal outcomes.

The consumption of this liquid becomes increasingly significant for extended periods of fasting, but can still provide benefits even during a 16-hour fasting window. The lengthier the period of fasting, the greater the impact on your digestive system and the more it will derive advantage from a prompt stimulation. However, it should be emphasized that deriving benefits from fasting does not require any of these aforementioned measures. Maintaining simplicity is crucial when embarking on your fasting journey, and in the event that this appears to be an overwhelming task, it is important to bear in mind that it is not obligatory; rather, it is an optional practice that provides additional advantages.

Solid food

Now, for eating. As previously mentioned, you may maintain your regular eating habits during a fast. But if you are interested in maximizing benefits, there are specific choices to ingest right after your fast ends that will work better to extend and promote the results of your fasting cycle.

Refrain from combining fats and carbohydrates, as the consumption of carbohydrates leads to the elevation of insulin levels, subsequently enhancing cellular receptivity. If your cells are receptive, fat will be stored when it is being consumed. After expending considerable effort in facilitating the reduction of adipose tissue through a vigorous process, this is the least desirable outcome. Consuming either fats or carbohydrates can be equally effective without any adverse consequences. Combine proteins with either fats or carbohydrates, but avoid pairing fats with carbohydrates.

Begin with a modest portion - For your inaugural meal, consider opting for a relatively compact serving size, if feasible. This indicates an approximate caloric intake of 500 to 600 calories. Your gastrointestinal system is still gradually increasing its activity, and inundating it with excessive intake all at once is not an optimal strategy. Consuming excessive amounts of food can potentially disrupt your digestive process, particularly after an extended period of fasting, leading to unintended overconsumption in the excitement of finally obtaining sustenance. Therefore, by engaging in premeditation and diligently managing the quantity, it will enhance the enjoyment and productivity of your fast.

Fluctuations in insulin levels - Endeavor to minimize the consumption of excessive carbohydrates during that initial meal. As previously stated, the consumption of carbohydrates results in insulin spikes, thereby rendering one's cells more receptive. Immediately following a period of abstaining from eating, it is not advisable to consume a considerable amount of carbohydrates. They can be tolerated in small quantities, but excessive consumption upon the conclusion of your fasting period is not advised.

Digestible foods are recommended as your digestive tract may be unaccustomed to processing food, and introducing something difficult to digest at once could potentially overwhelm your gastrointestinal system. This might be an incongruous moment to indulge in a substantial and succulent steak. Consider instead opting for delectable steamed vegetables in conjunction with a nutrient-rich source of dietary fats or an alternative that is conducive to maintaining a low glycemic index.

In consideration of all these regulations, it is imperative to note that as the duration of your fast increases, it becomes increasingly vital to remain mindful and gradually reintroduce food to your body. With intermittent fasting, the significance is somewhat diminished. However, should you embark upon an extended fast spanning three days or longer, the proper cessation of fasting assumes growing importance.

Intermittent fasting can be effortlessly practiced devoid of the inclusion of these supplementary regulations. As you delve deeper into the realm of fasting, you may discover that incorporating these suggestions enhances the benefits derived from your fasting endeavors. Just as one would select a fasting methodology, begin with a straightforward approach and progressively advance towards more intricate methods at a pace that aligns with your level of comfort.

The Fed State vs. The Significance of the Fasted State: An In-depth Examination

Your physique exists either in a state of being nourished or in a state of abstaining from nutrition. The preceding section emphasized this aspect. Let us carefully examine these two states.

The Fed State

This is the physical condition in which your body is placed upon consuming food, and subsequently engages in the processes of digestion, absorption, and assimilation of nutrients derived from the food you have ingested.

Under usual circumstances, the average American remains in a state of being well-nourished for the majority of the day. They would remain in this state throughout the entirety of the day, unless they refrain from eating when they fall asleep.

The Fasted State

This is the site where the phenomenon of effectively reducing persistent body fat and attaining weight loss is witnessed, alongside the manifold additional health advantages associated with adhering to an intermittent fasting regimen.

When an individual abstains from consuming calories for an extended duration, such as several hours, they induce their body to prioritize the utilization of stored body fat in order to sustain optimal functioning by continuously supplying the necessary energy. This inadvertently occurs for the majority of Americans during their sleep, albeit they inadvertently facilitate the body's access to glycogen upon awakening and proceeding towards the refrigerator.

The primary objective of intermittent fasting is to exercise control and purposefully regulate the designated period of fasting. This enables you to remain in the state of fasting, known as a state of enhanced lipid oxidation, for an extended duration.

The majority of schedules do not necessitate fasting for more than 18 hours, although there exist programs that entail a fasting period of 48 hours. Certainly, these programs provide you with the freedom to compensate for it by granting you unrestricted access to food for the subsequent 48 hours. However, the fundamental principle is as follows: in the event that one fasts for a duration of fewer than 24 hours, it can be deduced that fasting time frames should be allocated on a daily basis, thereby resulting in the existence of daily windows for consuming meals.

You will gradually implement the intermittent fasting program, taking it one day at a time, which will prove to be the optimal approach for you as a novice.

Let us examine a fundamental breakdown of IF schedules.

Suppose you have made the determination to adhere to a timetable that involves a 16-hour period of abstaining from food. Hence, it implies that you are confined to an eating window of 8 hours. If it is presumed that your schedule allows for an early initiation of the fasting period prior to retiring for the night, the omission of breakfast and elongation of the fast until approximately midday would enable the consumption of all meals within the designated time frame of 12 pm to 8 pm. Alternatively, if the fasting period concludes earlier, such as at 10 am, the subsequent period for eating would commence at 10 am and conclude at 6 pm.

This assertion does not imply that you dedicate the entirety of the 8-hour period to consuming food. It is imperative to uphold a sense of accountability as the ultimate objective is to achieve weight loss. Devise a strategic meal plan to align with the designated 8-hour timeframe. You have the option of selecting two meals in a large size, or six meals in a smaller size, or any other quantity that suits your preference. One advantageous aspect of intermittent fasting is the ability to select a method that aligns with one's individual preferences, so long as one remains committed to the prescribed timeframe. Following the completion of the 8-hour period, refrain from eating until the fasting period concludes.

Methods Of Practicing Intermittent Fasting: Various Approaches To Consider

To commence, when referring to "IF types", we are essentially indicating diverse forms of intermittent fasting programs, protocols, or schedules that can be adhered to. Alternatively, intermittent fasting is remarkably straightforward. Regardless of the specific program or schedule adhered to, one abstains from consuming food for a designated duration, followed by an allotted period for eating.

There exist numerous iterations of intermittent fasting protocols; however, the primary emphasis here will be on the most optimal ones tailored specifically to your needs, particularly at this juncture, as well as those that have demonstrated a verifiable history of success.

The 16/8 Method

To put it succinctly, the recommended approach involves observing a 16-hour fasting window followed by 8-hour period for consuming food.

This approach entails daily fasting periods lasting 14 to 16 hours, coupled with a limited eating window of 8-10 hours. The rationale behind the suggestion of a fasting duration between 14 to 16 hours is based on the recommendation for women to adhere to a 14-hour fasting window rather than a 16-hour window. This distinction is made considering that women exhibit more favorable responses to shorter periods of fasting.

This approach is commonly known as the Lean-gains protocol, and it gained widespread recognition due to the influence of Martin Berkhan, a well-regarded fitness enthusiast and expert.

This fasting approach is remarkably straightforward: it involves refraining from consuming any food beyond dinner and subsequently skipping breakfast the following day. For example, if you conclude your last meal of the day at 8pm, then you abstain from eating until 12pm the next day. By following this approach, you will effectively observe a fasting window of 16 hours between each meal. Initially, abstaining from breakfast may present certain challenges; however, you will quickly discern that the benefits far surpass the inconveniences.

Throughout the duration of your fasting phase, it is permissible to consume water, tea, coffee, or any other non-caloric beverages. Nevertheless, it is advisable to refrain from adding sugar to these beverages.

Indeed, if one's objective is weight loss through fasting, it is imperative to structure their dietary choices around wholesome and nutritious foods. Fasting for a duration of 16 hours appears to lose its purpose if it is subsequently followed by indulgence in unhealthy food choices. Losing weight while indulging in unhealthy foods poses a considerable challenge.

The 5:2 Diet

With the implementation of this protocol, it is required to observe a fasting period of 2 consecutive days within a week. The approach gained widespread recognition through the efforts of the British physician and journalist known as Michael Mosley.

This is yet another straightforward approach: you have the freedom to consume food according to your preferences for 5 days, while restricting your caloric intake to a minimal 600 calories per day on the remaining 2 days. This diet is well-suited for individuals who are reluctant to undergo daily fasting periods.

During days of fasting, it is advised that males consume 600 calories, whereas females are advised to consume 500 calories for optimal outcomes. Indeed, while the variances may appear slight, when observed over a substantial duration, the disparities become distinctively discernible.

An illustration of a 5:2 dietary pattern entails adhering to a routine in which one consumes a regular diet throughout the week, with the exception of Tuesdays and Thursdays. If one identifies as male, it is permissible to consume two meals consisting of 300 calories each on a designated fasting day. If you happen to identify as a female, it is advisable to consume two meals containing approximately 250 calories each during your days of fasting.

The Eat-Stop-Eat method

By adhering to this intermittent fasting regimen, you abstain from consuming any food for a duration of 24 hours either once or twice per week.

This approach was initially popularized by renowned fitness enthusiast and expert Brad Pilon, and has subsequently garnered significant acclaim and widespread acceptance. By abstaining from consuming meals from one evening until the following evening, the overall duration of fasting will encompass a full 24 hours.

Allow me to provide an illustration: Upon the completion of your dinner, specifically on a designated day such as Monday, you shall abstain from consuming any further sustenance until the subsequent dinner on Tuesday. By adhering to this practice, assuming you consistently arrange your meals to occur at identical intervals each day, you will have successfully accomplished a fast lasting for a full 24 hours. Nevertheless, you retain the flexibility to choose the manner in which you observe the fasting period: you can opt for a fast from morning until morning on the following day, or from noon to noon the next day. Regardless, the outcome will remain unchanged.

Throughout the designated period of fasting, individuals are permitted to consume non-caloric beverages such as water and coffee.

Considering your objective of weight loss, it is imperative that you adhere to a regular eating pattern on your non-fasting days. Specifically, it is crucial that you consume the usual quantity of food that you typically consume, without seeking to compensate for the fasting period.

One possible drawback lies in the arduous nature of a 24-hour fast, particularly for individuals lacking proficiency in fasting techniques. But you can work your way up from the 16/8 method, gradually increasing your fasted period until you are able to get to 24 hours.

Alternate Day Fasting

With the implementation of this fasting protocol, individuals abstain from consuming food on alternate days.

However, this particular approach is quite extreme, albeit there are various modifications available to mitigate its intensity. For individuals who are starting out, it is advisable to consume approximately 500 to 600 calories during fasting periods. Considering the fact that you will experience nights of going to bed without having eaten, it might be imperative to ensure adequate nourishment on the days allocated for meals. However, referring to this as an optimal technique for inexperienced individuals is challenging. If you possess a strong desire to effectively reduce body fat and possess the necessary emotional fortitude, I strongly encourage you to proceed and engage in that endeavor.

The warrior diet

In adherence to the warrior diet, the individual refrains from consuming food during daylight hours and engages in a substantial meal exclusively during the evening period.

One noteworthy aspect of this intermittent fasting approach is that you will not truly be abstaining from food for the entire day. It is unnecessary to do so, as you have the option to consume modest portions of vegetables and raw fruits during the day in order to sustain sufficient energy levels. This dietary plan is most effective when the eating window is constrained to a maximum duration of 4 hours. It is worth noting that allocating 4 hours for a single large meal should be ample time, considering that one does not typically require such an extensive period to consume a single serving."

Optimal outcomes can be attained by structuring your dietary regimen primarily around whole and minimally processed foods.

Guidelines And Strategies For Engaging In A Fast

Enduring extreme hunger poses significant challenges. Achieving success in modifying one's daily dietary habits while embracing a wholly new routine necessitates more than mere determination. You must be adequately prepared mentally to endure the challenges brought about by fasting, and possess the necessary discipline to adhere to the prescribed regulations.

There is no similarity between any two methods. Please bear in mind that the key factors for success in this endeavor lie in your psychological well-being, your level of readiness to endure the entirety of the task, and your unwavering commitment to accomplishing it with precision. In order to prevent the act of manipulating a pattern in order to accommodate your requirements, presented here are several suggestions and techniques to assist you in successfully excelling in your initial endeavor.

Know yourself

Fasting is not suitable for every individual. Fasting is not recommended for all individuals. Fasting may not be appropriate for everyone. Having made this statement, it is important to note that there are specific categories of individuals who should refrain from undertaking a fast. These demographics encompass expectant and lactating mothers, young children, and the elderly individuals. These cohorts consist of individuals with dietary needs that must be fulfilled. It is advised to consult with your physician, particularly if you are unwell or taking specific medications.

Know your method

Given your current state of good health, you should consider opting for a method that accommodates your schedule and aligns with your objectives. However, nothing is predefined. If you select a particular strategy and subsequently find that it is not suitable, simply modify your approach. Consider adopting a flexible approach as intermittent fasting does not necessitate strict adherence to a predetermined structure.

Stay hydrated

Ensuring optimal hydration is of utmost significance during the fasting period, particularly when engaging in resistance training. For gentlemen, it is advisable to consume up to 3 liters of water on days of fasting, while ladies are recommended to consume 2 liters per day. An additional advantageous aspect of this suggestion is that consuming water tends to reduce one's appetite.

Drink beverages

We have previously discussed the subject of water, however, the primary emphasis at this juncture pertains to tea and coffee. Consuming zero-calorie beverages such as black tea and coffee in the morning aids in suppressing appetite. Nonetheless, refrain from adding any sweetener as it is imperative to control calorie consumption.

Adhere to your fasting technique.

This advice holds utmost significance when it comes to achieving success in intermittent fasting. We are discussing the commitment to your meal and fasting regimen in question. It would be undesirable to shed 60 pounds, only to subsequently discover that one is unable to sustain commitment to their established regimen. In essence, you have discovered a valid rationale for your aversion towards fasting - its appeal has diminished.

Now, it is imperative that you refrain from further self-infliction of punitive measures. I typically emphasize to individuals that our primary objective is to derive enjoyment, cultivate a sense of self-satisfaction, and maintain enhanced physical well-being and longevity. However, it is imperative to ensure that intermittent fasting becomes an integral component of your lifestyle. Make necessary adaptations to your feeding and fasting schedule in order to ensure minimal disruption to various facets of your daily routine. Intermittent fasting is expected to enhance your productivity.

Please be mindful of your caloric intake.

Effective weight management primarily revolves around caloric intake regulation and the maintenance of a harmonious caloric equilibrium. If, like the majority of individuals, you seek the most efficient means to accomplish tasks, you are likely in search of a straightforward yet highly productive approach. You have the option to monitor your caloric intake either by manual tracking or by utilizing a mobile application. There exist several viable options at your disposal, provided that you locate the one that aligns most effectively with your needs.

The objective at hand is to maintain a caloric deficit ranging from 20 to 25 percent, which will result in a seemingly effortless weight loss. It is crucial to maintain honesty in recording one's progress and diligently track their Basal Metabolic Rate (BMR). If there is a lack of progress regarding your weight loss, it is essential to implement the appropriate modifications.

Have patience

It has been noted by someone that weight gain does not occur instantaneously, and therefore, one should not anticipate achieving a sculpted physique in just a few hours of following an intermittent fasting regimen. Practicing restraint is a critical factor in achieving weight loss and muscle development. It is imperative to adopt a realistic approach when setting your goals. Much like all facets of life, acquire the skill of commencing with modest endeavors and progressively expanding them. It is unrealistic to anticipate success in a highly competitive weight loss competition within a month's time, particularly considering your current weight surplus of one hundred pounds. Nevertheless, it is imperative that you maintain a sense of ambition. Establish well-defined objectives and commemorate every accomplishment along the way.

In conclusion, endeavor to engage in activities that occupy your time and accomplish tasks during the periods in which you are most efficient. This could potentially assist in diverting attention from food and effectively mitigating temptation. It is also imperative that you carefully monitor your dietary intake. Consuming a wide range of food items is a common practice, as you may be aware, contingent upon your intermittent fasting regimen. Do not employ the act of fasting as a means to rationalize consuming an excessive amount of unhealthy food. Always remember that your aim is to develop a lean and well-defined physique in a manner that promotes good health.

Potential Drawbacks Associated With Intermittent Fasting

Regrettably, nearly all things that possess advantages also come with corresponding drawbacks. In the realm of nutrition plans, IF is not exempt. Before undertaking an IF plan, it is imperative to consider certain drawbacks. Presented below are a few examples.

Full Compliance

Conformity to your plan is a prerequisite for IF. As an example, it is advised against breaching the fasting period by partaking in the consumption of soda or chewing gum. That is not deemed acceptable within the confines of IF. Complete adherence can consequently present a challenge that engenders discomfort for you.

Dreaded plateaus

Weight loss in the context of intermittent fasting also entails the potential occurrence of a plateau, akin to that experienced in various other weight loss strategies. The speed at which you are currently losing weight is approaching a threshold where further weight loss may become increasingly challenging. This phenomenon is commonly referred to as a weight plateau.

Bingeing

Numerous individuals succumb to the inclination of allowing their appetite and excitement to accumulate so much fervor that upon concluding the fasting period, their initial action is to indulgently consume and replenish their body with the very type of toxins they had just neutralized. This phenomenon is exclusively related to the realm of psychology, and if you possess a firm conviction that enduring extended periods of fasting would be profoundly challenging for you, it might be prudent to contemplate refraining from engaging in intermittent fasting.

Disruption of societal structure

Consumption of sustenance holds significant importance within the realm of human culture and society. We convene for formal gatherings encompassing various occasions, such as meetings, seminars, conferences, and diverse events, where thc presence of sustenance is highly probable. Omitting certain meals can result in an unbecoming appearance. Consider the scenario of attending a philanthropic event or a lavish banquet where participants are holding plates, while you find yourself standing or sitting in isolation, equipped only with a solitary water bottle. That has the potential to result in numerous explanations and uncomfortable situations. Moreover, the use of IF could potentially allude to a situation wherein one might frequently find themselves lacking in the enjoyment of late evening romantic meals, homemade familial suppers, celebratory birthday dinners, and convivial lunch gatherings.

Getting food-angry

According to a well-known proverb, a person who is hungry can become quite agitated, which is precisely why intermittent fasting may evoke strong emotions, leading to potential outbursts or increased irritability towards others as a result of hunger. Each individual responds to hunger in unique ways, and anger may manifest as one of the potential consequences of prolonged fasting.

Which individuals are advised to exercise caution or refrain from practicing intermittent fasting?

While it is indeed a commendable strategy, IF may not be suitable for everyone. Individuals who have a below-average body weight or a previous history of eating disorders should refrain from engaging in intermittent fasting (IF) without seeking appropriate consultations and medical guidance. It has the potential to be detrimental to their overall welfare. Furthermore, there exists some evidence suggesting that prolonged periods of food deprivation may exert a detrimental effect on women's fertility levels. The majority of these studies, however, have focused exclusively on rodents. Therefore, there is insufficient empirical evidence to definitively support the notion that women in their reproductive years should refrain from practicing intermittent fasting. Nonetheless, it is advisable to err on the side of caution.

Intermittent Fasting Procedure: The Warrior Diet

The Warrior Diet (WD) protocol is ideal for rule-followers or those who prefer lots of guidelines. This protocol is based on an alleged dietary pattern adopted by legendary ancient warriors who supposedly did not prefer the idea of consuming smaller meals multiple times a day. Warriors in ancient times consumed a maximum of 2 meals per day, as stated by Ori Hofmekler, the founder. The WD protocol necessitates fasting for 20 hours daily, leaving only 4 hours for eating.

The protocol is heavily criticized for being a fake form of intermittent fasting. Why? You can eat small due to the fasting period allowed in this protocol. For purist fasters, it's considered cheating and blasphemous. However, since your goal is effective and rapid weight loss, it shouldn't matter if it's a pure or mixed type of intermittent fasting. Many people see it as an effective way to lose weight through intermittent fasting. Case closed!

How to practice

Just consume necessary amounts of food within a 4-hour window daily, and fast for the remaining 20 hours. You can eat a large dinner followed by a small pre-bedtime meal right before fasting.

Eating the right food is the key to this diet, unlike the first 2 protocols. The protocol assumes that your body requires specific nutrients at night to align with your circadian rhythms. Humans are assumed to be wired to eat at night, not in the daytime, according to popular science. Similarly, you may consume small portions of uncooked vegetables, fruits, and lean protein, as previously stated. The protocol is primarily focused on eating below a specific threshold rather than completely abstaining from eating. The WD protocol aims to optimize your body's fight or flight response, leading to raised energy levels, heightened alertness, and improved metabolism, among other benefits.

The 4 hour eating phase is scheduled in the evening to aid in better digestion and allow your body to rest, relax, and recover with the help of the parasympathetic nervous system. Doing this also enables your body to effectively use the nutrients you consume for cell repair and heightened growth hormone production. Nighttime eating can enhance hormone production and improve fat-burning potential during daytime fasting.

The WD protocol, like the 2 earlier protocols, also emphasizes an eating order or sequence. Start with veggies, then consume fats and protein. If you're still hungry, consume additional fruit carbohydrates.

Advantages

While the fasting periods are long and daily, some people choose this protocol due to the allowance of small servings during the fasting window, making it more manageable. Many people who've followed this protocol experience increased fat burning and energy levels. As with the other protocols, the WD protocol allows you to improve your insulin sensitivity, which is key to promoting muscle mass growth and ultimately a faster metabolism or ability to burn body fat. Greater insulin sensitivity allows for higher carbohydrate tolerance. This enables your body to allocate nutrients more effectively to muscle and fat cells. Your body will be more efficient at utilizing protein for muscle growth. Improved insulin sensitivity reduces obesity and Type II diabetes risk.

The protocol also prevents the accumulation of excess energy. You can eat the perfect amount of calories for weight loss by simply tuning in to your body's signals of satisfaction. The human body is programmed to naturally deplete energy stores rather than replenish or build them up, as per the protocol's founder. Fasting enables regular depletion of energy stores. To fully optimize weight loss results, it is recommended to include a consistent exercise regimen alongside the other methods. Remember this. Hofmekler, the protocol's pioneer, states that losing weight is impacted more by nutritional stress than physical stress. First, prioritize getting the nutrition aspect correct. Adding regular exercise will enhance your weight loss benefits. The WD protocol can extend your quality of life. Hofmekler suggests that intermittent fasting, a form of nutritional stress, may extend lifespan for humans, animals, and bacteria. mTOR, also known as the mammalian target of rapamycin, is a protein essential for the survival, growth, and multiplication of healthy cells, as stated by him. It shaped you into the adult you are today.

This protein, while negative, remains crucial during adulthood. Hofmekler alleges it fosters superfluous growth in mature body parts. Managing premature aging, diabetes, and cancer risks requires reducing or inhibiting mTOR production. How can you accomplish that? Eating excessive amounts of food activates mTOR and consequently, starvation inhibits it. Intermittent fasting protocols like the Warrior Diet can reduce calories and lower risks for conditions, leading to a better and longer life.

Finally, the Warrior Diet is extremely easy to follow. If I find the concept of eating one large meal a day and multiple small portions of food daily to be difficult, then I am unsure about what simplicity truly means. The more simple it is, the fewer opportunities for errors.

Disadvantages

The Warrior Diet protocol may seem perfect with all its advantages. But it isn't. Like anything valuable, it has drawbacks. Thankfully, the quantity isn't significant. Admit it - a flexible fast, where you can snack on small portions, can be burdensome to constantly consider what and when to eat. The Lean Gains and Eat-Stop-Eat protocols are increasingly favored for this primary reason. And in addition to their practical aspects, the social aspects also need to be taken into account. If you're a social person, it'll be difficult to regularly meet friends due to the strict Warrior Diet. You must decide: lose weight and lose friends, or keep friends and keep weight. Your social life may be impacted if you commit to the WD protocol. If you're an introvert and rarely hang out with friends, this protocol won't be socially burdensome for you.

Another downside of the WD protocol is the requirement to completely fill yourself up for the remainder of the day. Fasting all day and consuming all required calories in one meal at night is extremely difficult, especially if you are used to a traditional 3-meals-a-day or 6-

small-frequent-meals diet. This transition is a significant change to make quickly. But you can solve the second challenge by slowly transitioning to the protocol. Allocate a fortnight to fully engage in the WD protocol. Gradually eat less food throughout the day and move that food to your dinner, until all or most of your daily intake is in your dinner.

Another approach is to consume high-calorie and filling foods such as virgin coconut oil or MCT oil to tackle the challenge of eating excessive amounts of food in a single sitting. You will feel less hungry at night by consuming less food. They also provide energy without impacting insulin sensitivity.

So Let's Do This Thing!

A how to guide

We aim to fast for 16 hours, 5 days a week. To fast, just refrain from eating for 16 hours, using any method you prefer. But it could be more challenging in practice.

Many believe they already fast 10-12 hours daily. But do they really? Most Americans don't provide their bodies with a 12 hour fasting period, despite the significant health benefits it offers according to studies. Think about it. After dinner, typically follows dessert or snacks, regardless of the time. Perhaps a snack before sleep or while watching television. What about beverages? Beer, wine, soda, hot tea with honey - all options available. All these require digestion.

Eat as you usually would initially. Maintain a log of your meals and their timings. Be very honest. No hurry, no stress. Our aim is to effectively and responsibly train our bodies and habits.

What is the maximum duration before your body requires digestion? You need to wait at least 8 hours before consuming more food or drinks. Refrain from consuming anything that needs to be digested during fasting to maintain its benefits. Fast for 10 hours, 3 days per week. Once you reach a point where you can do 10 hours without much difficulty, increase it to 12.

12 hours is significant to us. That is our bare minimum goal and actual starting position. Even at 12 hours, there is still benefit.

Digestion starts immediately when food enters your mouth. Saliva starts breaking down food. Food breaks down into tiny particles in your intestines for energy distribution in your body. Although there is more, we'll focus on this for now. Digestion, from beginning to end, lasts approximately 12 hours. After digestion, your body focuses on neglected projects. Your body can begin restoring homeostasis. It can return to its ideal equilibrium.

It's crucial to allow your body a minimum of 12 hours for this reason. Assuming you have accomplished it. You have reached the 12-hour mark. Continuing the fast beyond 12 hours every minute maintains the healing, fat burning balance in your body. The longer your body stays in homeostasis, the more fat burning benefits will accumulate. Attempt 13 hours biweekly, thrice, over a fortnight. Increase your fasting duration gradually by adding half an hour each day and taking necessary breaks.

Don't fear hunger. It won't cause any harm. If you have a habit of eating every few hours, this might be initially uncomfortable. Don't quit, even if you need to proceed at a slower pace. The advantages go well beyond just losing weight.

Before long, you'll effortlessly manage 16 hours without a second thought. You'll experience increased energy and appetite reduction, as well as noticeable physical changes within a few days.

At this juncture, choices are available. You can either attempt a 24-hour fast if you feel good, maintain the same approach, or opt for an 18/6 fast with a 6-hour feeding window.

Take time off, regardless of your choice. No difference in benefits between intermittent fasting 5 days a week and 7 days a week. So don't. Allocate at least two days per week (or even three) for communal meals with loved ones. Do it, if you want to go out for drinks a few nights a week. Late night pizza party? Agreed! Having two days off a week promotes mental well-being and prevents burnout, while also providing benefits. During that lenient period, a substantial meal with carbs aids in restoring glycogen, maintaining a high metabolism, and elevating leptin levels. To sustain fat burning, maintain high leptin levels, as it is the key hormone responsible.

Enjoy yourself, but remember the calorie in calorie out rule while doing so. A continuous gummy bear party lasting for 16 hours is likely not the wisest choice.

The 16/8 Method

Try a 24-hour fasting routine with an eating window of 8 hours and a fasting window of 16 hours, known as the 16/8 method. This involves alternating periods of fasting and eating within a specific time frame. Eat only during an 8-hour window, such as 12 pm to 8 pm, and fast for the remaining 16 hours.

NOTE:

Choose early morning for feeding as metabolism and energy burning capacity are highest then. Choose nutritious foods and calorie-free drinks like black coffee, tea, and herbal tea while fasting for 16 hours.

Pros

Research has found that the 16/8 method is easy to follow, according to study participants. Krista Varady, an associate kinesiology and nutrition professor at the University of Illinois,

Chicago, led one of these studies. Fewer participants quit the 16/8 diet compared to other fasting diets, as per the study.

No need for calorie counting with the 16/8 method, like other intermittent fasting diets. You don't feel intense hunger like in full day fasts.

Cons

Most people following the 16/8 diet skip evening meals, which can be problematic. Skipping evening meals affects your social and home life.

Once more, this approach imposes a limited timeframe. Eating within a limited time frame promotes a dieting mentality. If you consistently believe you are adhering to a diet, your inclination to sustain the approach over time will diminish.

Alternate-Day Fasting

On this intermittent fasting plan, you alternate fasting and unrestricted eating days. So, you will restrict your food for half of the time.

You can consume calorie-free beverages like black coffee, water, and tea on your fasting days. It's that easy. You can choose to follow a modified ADF approach, consuming around 500 calories on fasting days or 20-25% of your energy needs. The health benefits are the same, regardless of whether you consume the fasting day calories during dinner, lunch, or in small increments throughout the day.

Pros

Alternate day fasting has been proven to not significantly increase compensatory hunger compared to continuous calorie restriction. After a couple of weeks, individuals following intermittent fasting claim their hunger disappears, making fasting days effortless.

Cons

Compensatory hunger is a drawback of alternate-day fasting. It is extreme hunger caused by calorie restriction, leading to overeating when you finally allow yourself to eat.

ADF can be challenging to maintain alongside gym workouts. Being exhausted can hinder your ability to exercise effectively. This leads some individuals to intentionally skip their exercise sessions.

The Warrior Diet

You will need to spend most of your day either eating very little or fasting, and then consume a big meal in the evening. Exercise is required with intermittent fasting, as it is based on the warrior diet concept where ancient warriors ate minimally or fasted during the day due to their active lifestyle. They would subsequently cook and consume one evening meal.

So, if you choose to follow this diet, expect to eat very little for approximately 20 hours each day. You may have fluids and certain snacks if hunger becomes unbearable during the initial stages of fasting. Refer to the final chapter for further details about the meals.

Choose nutritious meals with plenty of vegetables to stay satisfied without overeating.

Pros

Most people consider this method the best for weight loss. Empty stomach morning workouts lead to more weight loss than exercising after eating. The diet will provide you with a continuous flow of fat burning hormones in your blood for approximately six to eight hours each day. Experts say the ketogenic diet is likely the only one with a comparable effect.

Additionally, the warrior diet's efficacy is enhanced by the overeating phase, which stimulates a significant thermic effect, resulting in increased calorie expenditure during the process of food digestion and absorption. During the overeating phase, your body expends numerous calories digesting the large amount of food consumed.

Adopting the warrior diet and exercising enhances muscle growth. Exercising while under-eating can enhance muscle growth during resistance training. Scientists support fasting training to boost muscle-building genes.

Cons

Some people can exercise on an empty stomach, while others cannot. Long periods of fasting may cause dizziness, dehydration, fatigue, and impair performance, especially during workouts with limited fuel. You may also encounter risks from low blood sugar, specifically hypoglycemia.

Also, a single meal is unlikely to provide all the necessary nutrients for good health. Obtaining all essential nutrients in one large meal is extremely challenging. You need to eat several meals daily for your body to obtain necessary nutrients, just like most people.

Additionally, a pattern of minimal daytime eating followed by nighttime overeating can cause a significant rise in blood sugar after your evening meal and subsequently lead to a sharp decrease in blood sugar levels during periods of no food intake. This eating method is not advisable as it raises your risk of developing diseases.

You can choose the suitable intermittent fasting method by using the knowledge you gained about popular methods. The next chapter will discuss nutrition for optimal weight loss during intermittent fasting, as making healthier food choices is important for overall health.

Intermittent Fasting Has A Provenance

Various diets and eating regimes have become increasingly popular in the industrialized world for decades. Health and fitness programs have also been extensive and impressive. Both these recent occurrences have arisen due to a significant rise in obesity levels and a widespread epidemic of overweight individuals. Around 66% of Western populations are overweight and obese individuals face a sevenfold increased risk of premature death. Moreover, countries previously afflicted by malnutrition have swiftly embraced the Western diet, resulting in a growing prevalence of obesity.

Conventional diets are ineffective, as indicated by this. Studies indicate that, typically, individuals regain lost weight within five years of initiating a diet, and approximately 40% end up gaining more weight than their initial starting point. Amidst this peculiar paradox, people seek thinness as an ideal, turning to mannequins and actors as their body shape icons. Girls under the age of ten are highly susceptible to this behavior, with 80% of American girls trying various diets in pursuit of their desired body shape. Girls who diet when young tend to binge eat later on.

We should be concerned not only about the weight gain and desires of our youth. Obesity leads to various health issues like eating disorders, low self-esteem, and diverse types of cancer. Excessive body fat is consistently linked to the prevalent issue of increasing rates of type 2 diabetes, making it the primary health concern in many nations. This type of diabetes, once rare, is now considered a major global social health risk and is frequently referred to as a ticking health bomb.

Dietary science often becomes unreliable over time. Eggs were once thought to raise cholesterol levels, but now we know that the cholesterol in eggs is actually beneficial. Our current dietary recommendations may change from promoting high grain and carbohydrate intake to advocating for increased consumption of saturated fats in the future. The dietary advice is complex, and there are concerns due to diet experts profiting from promoting new diets and related products. It's hard to tell if the advice we receive benefits us or the advice-givers, given the potential for massive profits. The global population appears to become increasingly obese and less healthy.

We must acknowledge the need to reconsider our eating habits. Maybe the solution isn't in a trendy diet that requires constant willpower and calorie tracking. The path to wellness may involve more than just our diet and commitment to exercise. Reflecting on our past provides an alternate path forward.

Fasting dates back thousands of years. We have fasted due to either voluntary decisions or limited alternatives, throughout our evolutionary past. Our bodies have evolved to tolerate extended periods without food. Recent food availability changes contribute to weight gain and declining health.

All major religions support fasting as evidence for its benefits. Hippocrates, Plato, Aristotle, and Socrates endorsed fasting for mental clarity and physical well-being. Animals stop eating when sick. Many of us have ancestors who recall times of scarce food and deprivation. They witnessed a time when the majority of people were slender. Today, a significant portion of the population is obese and there is a possibility that, for the first time ever, our children may have shorter lifespans than their parents. Maybe we should consider returning to our historical dietary practices.

The Fundamental Tenets Of Intermittent Fasting

When the majority of individuals contemplate intermittent fasting, they typically envision abstaining from their preferred meals and undergoing a state of extreme hunger. This does not align with the core principles and purpose of fasting. It has been ingrained in us that we must consistently consume food in copious amounts, as any lapse in doing so may have detrimental effects on our physical well-being. On the contrary, the inverse holds true. Our physical structures possess far greater resilience than we often acknowledge, and on occasion, they necessitate respite from excessive nourishment.

Intermittent fasting revolves around establishing an equilibrium wherein one alternates between designated periods of nourishment and periods of refraining from food. It does not necessitate adherence to a rigorous dietary regimen, rather, the emphasis lies on the designated periods during which one should consume food. The timing, rather than the content, is the crucial factor.

Intermittent fasting is intended to accommodate your individual timetable. The strategies that prove effective for others may not invariably yield the same results for you. Considering the fact that you naturally undergo a fasting period of eight hours while you are asleep, it would be advisable to prolong this fasting window for a slightly longer duration. Therefore, it is recommended to forgo breakfast and commence your first meal at noon. You will subsequently partake in your evening meal around eight o'clock. Intermittent fasting involves the adoption of cycles comprising periods of both feasting and fasting, wherein one divides their day or week accordingly.

The aforementioned proposition is frequently denoted as the 16/8 method. One adheres to a fasting period of 16 hours, followed by an eating window that spans eight hours. Although it may appear torturous, the process is surprisingly straightforward and yields a surprising surge of energy beyond one's expectations. In the initial phase, it typically requires approximately one week for the body to acclimate to the modified eating pattern. However, subsequent adherence to the established regimen will seamlessly become effortless and instinctive.

It is crucial to bear in mind that while observing the fasting cycle, it is imperative to ensure adequate hydration with water or tea, while refraining from consuming any form of sugar. One must refrain from consuming any food products or dietary supplements that contain calories.

The Comparison between Dietary Restrictions and Intermittent Fasting

The majority of individuals adhere to specific dietary regimens. The media has effectively promoted diets as the optimal approach for achieving weight loss, building lean muscle, and attaining a state of good health. If the efficacy of dieting is indeed substantial, what accounts for the escalating incidence of lifestyle diseases? Why is it that individuals are not achieving the weight loss results as assured by their fitness mentors and health professionals?

Dieting represents a temporary and artificial solution to an underlying issue. One embarks on a dietary regimen solely with the aim of achieving immediate, targeted outcomes, without harboring any intention of adhering to it in perpetuity. Once you have successfully attained your objectives, there is a strong likelihood that you will regress into your prior detrimental habits. Intermittent fasting entails the adherence to designated time periods within a day for the consumption of calories, thereby constituting a natural process. Refrain from caloric consumption during the designated fasting period. It boasts enhanced long-term maintainability and can swiftly be embraced as a way of life.

It is imperative that we abandon this misconception that adhering to a six-meal paradigm is essential for maintaining good health. Consider the following perspective: As the human body undergoes the process of digestion, it expends calories and employs energy. As you allocate additional time to the act of consuming food, the body's duration of calorie expenditure proportionally extends. Upon initial examination, it may appear favorable, although that assertion is unfounded. Your physical being finds itself ensnared in an unceasing process that drains energy and receives scarcely adequate repose for self-renewal. Hence, it is more advantageous to facilitate calorie burning within a limited timeframe as opposed to over the course of the entire day.

A dietary regimen enables individuals to diminish the quantity of food consumed during each meal; however, how many individuals possess the ability to accurately ascertain the precise amount of food necessitated per meal for the purpose of weight loss? Furthermore, assuming one possesses the capacity to accomplish this task, how many individuals possess the level of discipline required to adhere to such a course of action? Diets often stipulate the permissible food options one can consume. Contrarily, intermittent fasting does not center around limiting the quantity or the varieties of food one can ingest. The objective is to effectively regulate your hunger while simultaneously reaping the enduring advantages of fasting.

Scientists have made a revelation that reducing the frequency of meals within a condensed time frame results in more significant weight loss compared to consuming smaller meals throughout the day and facing the challenge of calorie counting.

The argument being made is that dieting, being a short-term endeavor characterized by stress and a high likelihood of failure, lacks the potential health benefits associated with intermittent fasting. Individuals frequently transition in and out of dietary regimens, resulting in the subsequent reversal of the progress they had previously achieved. Your physiological response to a traditional dietary regimen is inclined to resist and actively counteract your endeavors to lose weight. Nevertheless, intermittent fasting is a innate approach that the body effortlessly acclimates to, as it thrives when it alternates between periods of indulgence and abstaining.

Approach 4: The Warrior Diet

Ori Hefmekler, an individual who transitioned from a military background to become a distinguished fitness professional and accomplished author, pioneered this methodology in the year 2001.

How it works

This particular fasting approach possesses distinctiveness and provokes debate within the community. Firstly, it is the singular approach that lacks empirical evidence. This technique was exclusively devised by Ori Hofmekler, drawing inspiration solely from his military experiences. Furthermore, he obtained some of his insights through a comprehensive analysis of historical cultures such as Rome and Sparta.

He made note of the fact that soldiers of antiquity consumed minimal amounts of food throughout the day, opting instead to partake in a single substantial meal come evening. Based on this observation, he arrived at the conclusion that this was the intended manner of eating prior to the advent of modernity. According to his argument, consumption in this manner stimulates the innate survival mechanisms of the human body.

According to this approach, it is necessary to observe a 20-hour fasting period and consume a single substantial meal during a 4-hour timeframe in the evening, alternating on a daily basis. According to the inventor's terminology, the period of fasting for 20 hours is known as the "under-eating phase," whereas the 4-hour period is designated as the "under-eating phase."

For whom is it most suitable?

As a result of the stringent regulations associated with this approach, it may not be suitable for all individuals.

This approach is most suitable for individuals who possess a strong inclination towards adhering to rules and encompass a high level of self-discipline. This phenomenon arises due to the inherent propensity of this approach to honor its designated appellation. To ensure your survival with this method, it is imperative that you embrace a lifestyle akin to that of a warrior.

How to do it

"If you possess unwavering confidence in your suitability for this technique, the subsequent instructions delineate the course of action for its implementation:

Initially, establish a strategy for the nourishment you intend to consume throughout the period of restricted caloric intake. The originator of this methodology advocates for moderate portions of fruits, vegetables, and protein. These provisions are intended to stimulate the body's inherent fight or flight mechanism. This serves the purpose of maintaining bodily alertness and facilitating fat-burning processes.

Furthermore, devise a comprehensive meal schedule for the period of excessive consumption. It is advisable to commence with a combination of vegetables, protein, and fat. Subsequently, should you continue to experience hunger, you may consume a portion of carbohydrates. The objective of consuming such foods is to facilitate bodily relaxation, as well as to support both tranquility and healthy digestion. They also assist in the process of repair and growth.

Once steps 1 and 2 have been carefully deliberated, proceed to establish a weekly timetable and commence its implementation. I would suggest commencing at the commencement of the week, as doing so facilitates the monitoring and adherence to your designated timetable.

If an individual possesses a steadfast determination and assertiveness, the Warrior diet can indeed prove to be efficacious.

Are you enthusiastic about acquiring further knowledge? Continue reading to discover an additional fasting approach that proves highly effective.

Health Risks Of Fasting

Intermittent fasting has rapidly garnered attention within the wellness community, as its remarkable impacts on health are being widely discussed. According

According to a number of scientific studies, it possesses the capacity to facilitate weight reduction, diminish the likelihood of cancer and other ailments,

and potentially extend your life expectancy. Nonetheless, there is a prevalent argument which asserts that intermittent fasting is potentially unsafe and

suitable for a ll. It is advisable to refrain from practicing intermittent fasting.

if:

One must strive to avoid experiencing sensations of hunger, fatigue, dehydration, or irritability.

This form of fasting is certainly unsuitable for individuals lacking fortitude. Despite the absence of health concerns on your part,

will undoubtedly encounter certain unfavorable side effects, such as a rumbling stomach and discomfort.

exhaustion.

You are susceptible to developing eating disorders.

There is a notable association between intermittent fasting and bulimia nervosa. Hence, people

Individuals who possess a predisposition towards eating disorders should refrain from engaging in any form of fasting. The presence of a familial history of eating disorders along with tendencies towards impulsive behavior are notable risk factors.

factors for developing eating disorders.

16

You require significant caloric intake.

Amongst the individuals who have a requirement for high consumption

Individuals who typically require higher caloric intake on a daily basis are pregnant women, lactating mothers, and individuals with elevated nutritional needs.

are experiencing a low body weight and encountering challenges in achieving weight gain.

You are experiencing specific medical conditions,

such as diabetes

It is imperative for individuals and groups of concern to refrain from practicing intermittent fasting, particularly without prior consultation with their healthcare provider, as it may pose potential hazards.

to their wellbeing. Those with diabetes and individuals who are underweight fall into this category. Individuals with any pre-existing health conditions

Individuals with underlying health conditions should carefully reconsider the option of fasting and consult with their healthcare professional prior to any dietary changes.

changes.

Intermittent fasting necessitates abstaining from food for consecutive days, a practice that can ultimately enhance the insulin sensitivity of your body. Insulin sensitivity is

Undeniably advantageous, as it facilitates optimal cellular energy utilization derived from ingested nourishment, leading to significant overall benefits.

Your blood sugar levels become more manageable. Nevertheless, hunger and hypoglycemia

Sugar leads to heightened physiological stress in the body. P rolonged

17

Abstaining from food, leading to heightened stress levels and decreased blood sugar, can have adverse effects on your health.

hormones.

A multitude of studies have provided evidence that

Intermittent fasting offers a multitude of exceptional advantages. may be, caution must still be exercised."

When it comes to intermittent fasting, it is essential to note that

Please keep in mind that a significant portion of the research has been carried out on

unfortunately, hampering our comprehension of

It could be applicable to the human species. According to information provided by Harvard Health,

Additionally, various empirical investigations have been conducted on human subjects.

Nevertheless, these investigations have been undertaken on...

limited clusters of individuals, leading to the resultant discoveries

may not be applicable to a significant portion of the population.

The safety and potential of intermittent fasting

"complications exhibit variability based on the unique characteristics of each individual and multiple health factors such as pre-existing medical conditions

circumstances, sex, way of life, overall health, and age. Please be advised that it is necessary to consult with a medical professional prior to making any substantial alterations to your dietary habits.

www.ingramcontent.com/pod-product-compliance
Lightning Source LLC
Chambersburg PA
CBHW071213020426
42333CB00015B/1389